VIKAS CHAUHAN

Top 5 Ageless Vitality Tips

Secrets to Lifelong Health and Wellness

This book was professionally typeset on Reedsy.
Find out more at reedsy.com

Contents

1

Introduction

In the quest for a life filled with energy, health, and happiness, the concept of ageless vitality emerges as a beacon of promise. It speaks to the possibility of living fully at any age, with a spirit undimmed by the passing years and a body that thrives with wellness. Top 5 Ageless Vitality Tips is not just about extending our lifespan but enriching the quality of every moment we live. It's a commitment to nurturing ourselves in ways that transcend conventional boundaries of age, tapping into the timeless essence of our being to unlock a reservoir of vitality that is both enduring and transformative.

At its core, this book is an invitation to embark on a journey of self-discovery and holistic well-being. It challenges us to rethink our perceptions of aging, to see beyond the chronological markers and societal expectations, and to envision a life where vitality is continuously renewed and preserved. This journey is grounded in the understanding that vitality is the result of harmony between the body, mind, and spirit—a harmony that can be cultivated through mindful nutrition, regular physical activity, restorative sleep, mental resilience, and meaningful social connections.

This book is both personal and universal, reflecting individual aspirations for health and well-being while also drawing on collective wisdom and scientific insights. It recognizes that the path to vitality is unique for each person, shaped by individual circumstances, preferences, and challenges. Yet, it also underscores the commonalities that bind us in our pursuit of a vibrant life—our shared desire for happiness, our innate capacity for resilience, and our profound connection to the world around us.

This introduction to ageless vitality is not merely an overview of principles and practices; it is a call to action. It invites you to engage deeply with the essence of vitality, to explore the multifaceted dimensions of well-being, and to commit to a lifestyle that fosters longevity and joy. Through the pages that follow, you will discover the building blocks of ageless vitality, learn practical strategies for integrating these principles into your life, and be inspired by the transformative potential of embracing vitality at any age.

This book is a testament to the power of intention, the beauty of growth, and the enduring strength of the human spirit. It's a journey toward a life not just lived, but lived well, with every day an opportunity to renew our commitment to vitality, to deepen our understanding of wellness, and to celebrate the infinite possibilities that arise when we choose to live with purpose and passion.

Welcome to the journey of ageless vitality—a journey that begins with a promise to yourself to live every moment with energy, health and happiness.

2

Nourishing Foundations: Unlocking the Secrets of Anti-Aging Nutrition

Introduction to Anti-Aging Nutrition

The quest for ageless vitality is as much about the spirit as it is about the body and at the heart of this journey lies nutrition—a powerful, yet often misunderstood, tool in our arsenal against aging. The foods we consume do more than just fuel our daily activities; they provide the essential building blocks for our cells, influence our hormonal balance, and interact with our genetic blueprint in ways that can significantly impact our health, longevity, and vitality.

The Influence of Nutrition on Aging and Vitality

Nutrition plays a pivotal role in aging and vitality, acting through mechanisms that affect every aspect of our biological functioning. Antioxidants, found abundantly in fruits and vegetables, combat oxidative stress—one of the primary culprits in cellular aging and the development of chronic diseases. Omega-3 fatty acids, sourced from fish and plant oils, are crucial for maintaining cell membrane integrity and reducing inflammation, a key factor in aging and metabolic health. Meanwhile, dietary fibers support digestive health and modulate the body's use of sugars, helping to control weight and reduce the risk of diabetes. Each nutrient, each bite, contributes to a complex interplay that can either accelerate or decelerate the aging process, influencing our vitality from the cellular level up.

Debunking Common Myths About Diet and Aging

Myth 1: Aging inevitably leads to decline, and diet can't change that. Reality: While aging is a natural process, the rate and manner in which we age are profoundly influenced by our diets. Nutrient-rich, balanced diets have been shown to mitigate the risk of many age-related diseases, improve mental and physical function, and enhance quality of life, even in later years.

Myth 2: High-fat foods are always bad for you. Reality: The type of fat matters more than the amount. Unsaturated fats, such as those found in avocados, nuts, and olive oil, can protect against heart disease and improve brain health, while trans fats and excessive saturated fats should be avoided.

Myth 3: Supplements can replace a healthy diet. Reality: While supplements can help fill nutritional gaps, they cannot replicate the complex mix of nutrients and phytochemicals found in whole foods. A diet based on a variety of whole foods is essential for promoting health and longevity.

Myth 4: It's too late to change your diet and improve your health. Reality: It's never too late to make dietary changes that can significantly impact your vitality and longevity. Regardless of age, switching to a nutrient-rich diet can improve heart health, cognitive function, and overall well-being.

In embracing the power of anti-aging nutrition, we unlock the potential not just for a longer life, but for a richer, more vibrant existence. By choosing foods that nourish and sustain, we set the stage for a journey of health that can defy the expectations of aging, proving that vitality knows no age limit.

The Science of Nutrition and Longevity

The intricate dance between nutrition and longevity is a testament to the profound impact that diet can have on our health and lifespan. At the core of this relationship arc key nutrients that play vital roles in maintaining health and preventing age-related decline. Understanding these nutrients, and how they work in harmony within our bodies, offers a blueprint for a diet that not only extends life but enriches it with vitality.

Key Nutrients and Their Roles

- **Antioxidants (Vitamins C and E, Selenium, and Beta-Carotene):** These powerful compounds combat oxidative stress by neutralizing free radicals, molecules that can damage cells and contribute to aging and diseases, including cancer and heart disease. Foods rich in antioxidants, such as berries, nuts, and leafy greens, are essential for cellular health and longevity.
- **Omega-3 Fatty Acids:** Found in fatty fish, flaxseeds, and walnuts, omega-3s are crucial for brain health, reducing inflammation, and lowering the risk of heart disease. Their role in maintaining cell membrane integrity also supports overall cellular function and health.
- **Fiber:** A key player in digestive health, fiber found in whole grains, fruits, and vegetables helps regulate blood sugar

levels, supports heart health, and is linked with a lower risk of several chronic diseases. Additionally, fiber supports a healthy gut microbiome which is crucial for immune function and inflammation control.

- **Calcium and Vitamin D:** These nutrients work in tandem to support bone health, crucial for preventing osteoporosis and maintaining mobility in older age. While calcium is found in dairy products, leafy greens, and fortified foods, Vitamin D can be synthesized through sunlight exposure and is also found in fatty fish and fortified foods.
- **Polyphenols:** Present in foods like dark chocolate, green tea, and red wine, polyphenols have been shown to reduce inflammation and lower the risk of several diseases. Their role in longevity is linked to their antioxidant properties and their ability to modulate risk factors for chronic diseases.

Core Principles of Anti-Aging Nutrition

The journey towards ageless vitality is underpinned by core principles that guide our dietary choices. Among these, the emphasis on whole foods over processed, the pursuit of balance and variety, and the importance of proper hydration stand out as foundational pillars. These principles not only support longevity but also enhance the quality of life, ensuring that our bodies are nourished, protected, and primed for optimal functioning.

Whole Foods Over Processed

The preference for whole, unprocessed foods is a cornerstone of anti-aging nutrition. Whole foods, such as fruits, vegetables, whole grains, nuts, seeds, and lean proteins, are minimally altered from their natural state, retaining their full spectrum of nutrients, including vitamins, minerals, fiber, and antioxidants. These nutrients work synergistically to support cellular health, reduce inflammation, and protect against oxidative stress and DNA damage, which are key factors in aging and the development of chronic diseases.

In contrast, processed foods often contain added sugars, unhealthy fats, and artificial ingredients, while lacking in essential nutrients. Regular consumption of processed foods has been linked to increased risks of obesity, heart disease, diabetes, and other age-related conditions. By choosing whole foods, we provide our bodies with the nourishment needed to thrive, promoting longevity and vitality.

Balance and Variety

A varied diet rich in vitamins, minerals, and antioxidants is crucial for covering the broad spectrum of nutrients our bodies require. Each nutrient plays a unique role in maintaining health and preventing disease; for example, vitamin D and calcium are essential for bone health, while omega-3 fatty acids support brain function and reduce inflammation. A diet that includes a wide range of colorful fruits and vegetables, whole grains, lean proteins, and healthy fats ensures that we receive a diverse array of these nutrients.

Balance and variety also prevent nutritional deficiencies and reduce the risk of chronic diseases, while making meals more enjoyable and satisfying. Incorporating a rainbow of foods into your diet not only maximizes nutrient intake but also introduces different flavors and textures, making healthy eating a pleasurable experience.

Proper Hydration

Water is the elixir of life, playing a critical role in every cellular process in our bodies. It aids in digestion, absorption of nutrients, circulation, and detoxification, helping to flush toxins from our system and support cellular health. Proper hydration is essential for maintaining the balance of bodily fluids, regulating body temperature, and ensuring the proper functioning of our organs.

Moreover, staying adequately hydrated can improve skin elasticity, reducing the appearance of fine lines and wrinkles, and contribute to a more youthful complexion. It also supports cognitive function and energy levels, both of which are vital for maintaining quality of life as we age.

In summary, the core principles of anti-aging nutrition—prioritizing whole foods over processed, embracing balance and variety, and ensuring proper hydration—form the foundation of a diet that supports longevity and vitality. By adhering to these principles, we can nourish our bodies at the deepest levels, promoting health and well-being throughout the lifespan.

Superfoods for Ageless Vitality

In the quest for ageless vitality, certain foods stand out for their remarkable nutrient profiles and anti-aging properties. Dubbed "superfoods," these nutritional powerhouses are rich in antioxidants, vitamins, minerals, and other compounds that can help slow the aging process and bolster health. Incorporating these superfoods into your diet can be a delicious and effective way to enhance your longevity and vitality.

Detailed Exploration of Superfoods

- **Berries (Blueberries, Strawberries, Raspberries):** Berries are loaded with antioxidants, such as vitamin C and anthocyanins which protect against oxidative stress and inflammation, key drivers of aging. They also offer fiber and vitamins that support heart health and brain function.

- **Leafy Greens (Spinach, Kale, Swiss Chard):** These vegetables are high in vitamins A, C, E, and K, along with minerals like calcium and iron. They contain potent antioxidants that can protect vision, reduce the risk of chronic diseases, and promote skin health.
- **Nuts and Seeds (Almonds, Walnuts, Chia Seeds):** Rich in healthy fats, protein, and fiber, nuts and seeds are excellent for heart health and weight management. They also contain antioxidants and minerals that support brain health and reduce inflammation.
- **Fatty Fish (Salmon, Mackerel, Sardines):** A prime source of omega-3 fatty acids, fatty fish are crucial for maintaining brain health, reducing inflammation, and supporting cardiovascular health. There are vegetarian sources available for omega-3.
- **Green Tea:** Known for its high levels of catechins, green tea is a powerful antioxidant that can protect against cellular damage, support healthy aging, and aid in weight management.
- **Dark Chocolate (at least 70% cocoa):** Besides being a delicious treat, dark chocolate is rich in flavonoids that can improve heart health, increase blood flow, and reduce inflammation.
- **Avocados:** Packed with healthy monounsaturated fats, fiber, and potassium, avocados support heart health, healthy aging, and can help maintain healthy cholesterol levels.
- **Turmeric:** This spice contains curcumin, a compound

with strong anti-inflammatory and antioxidant properties, making it beneficial for reducing the risk of chronic diseases and supporting cognitive function.

Practical Tips on Incorporating These Foods into Daily Meals

1. **Start with Breakfast:** Add berries to your morning oatmeal, yogurt or smoothie. Sprinkle chia seeds or ground flaxseeds for a nutrient boost.
2. **Snack Smart:** Keep a stash of mixed nuts and seeds for a healthy snack. Pair dark chocolate with almonds for an afternoon treat that satisfies and provides antioxidant benefits.
3. **Greens with Every Meal:** Aim to include a serving of leafy greens in every meal, whether it's a spinach salad at lunch, kale added to a smoothie, or Swiss chard sautéed as a dinner side dish.
4. **Opt for Omega-3:** Chia pudding, Flaxseed smoothie, Quinoa salad, Walnut and Date Balls or baking mackerel with herbs and lemon.
5. **Sip on Green Tea:** Replace your morning coffee with green tea or enjoy it as a refreshing afternoon drink. It's hydrating and packed with antioxidants.
6. **Spice It Up:** Add turmeric to soups, stews, or rice dishes. Mixing turmeric with black pepper can enhance the absorption of curcumin.
7. **Avocado Everywhere:** Use avocado as a spread on whole-grain toast, add it to salads, or blend it into smoothies for a creamy texture and a dose of healthy fats.

Incorporating these superfoods into your daily meals doesn't have to be complicated. With a little creativity and planning, you can enjoy the myriad benefits they offer, paving the way for a life filled with vitality and longevity.

Overcoming Common Nutritional Challenges

Adopting and maintaining a diet that supports ageless vitality can be challenging, especially when faced with common obstacles such as busy schedules, dietary restrictions, and budget constraints. However, with strategic planning and a few practical tips, these barriers can be navigated successfully, allowing for a nutritious diet that promotes longevity and well-being.

Addressing Busy Schedules

Plan Ahead: Dedicate time each week to plan your meals. This can help ensure that you have a healthy option available, reducing the temptation to opt for fast food or processed meals.

Batch Cooking: Prepare and cook meals in batches during your free time. Store portions in the fridge or freezer for a quick and easy meal on busy days.

Healthy Snacks: Keep a stock of healthy snacks, such as nuts, fruits, and yogurt, for those times when you need a quick bite. These can prevent hunger and provide you with essential nutrients without the need for extensive preparation.

Navigating Dietary Restrictions

Research and Substitute: For those with dietary restrictions, research alternative sources of essential nutrients. For example, if you're lactose intolerant, almond milk or soy milk can be good sources of calcium and vitamin D.

Consult a Professional: Consider consulting a dieticians or nutritionist. They can offer personalized advice and help you design a diet that meets your nutritional needs despite restrictions.

Managing Budget Constraints

Buy in Bulk: Purchase non-perishable items like whole grains, legumes, and nuts in bulk. These items are often cheaper in larger quantities and can be stored for a long time.

Seasonal and Local: Opt for fruits and vegetables that are in season and locally produced. They are usually more affordable and fresher, providing more nutrients.

Minimize Waste: Plan your meals to use all the ingredients you buy. Use leftovers creatively to ensure that food is not wasted and your budget is maximized.

By implementing these strategies, you can overcome common nutritional challenges and support your journey towards ageless vitality. Remember, the key to a nutritious diet is consistency and balance, not perfection. Making small, sustainable changes over time can lead to significant benefits for your health and longevity.

Supplements: Do You Need Them?

In the quest for ageless vitality, supplements often emerge as a topic of interest and debate. While a well-balanced diet is the cornerstone of good health, there are circumstances where supplements can play a supportive role. However, it's crucial to approach supplementation with a balanced perspective, understanding both its benefits and limitations.

The Role of Supplements in an Anti-Aging Diet

Supplements can fill nutritional gaps in your diet, especially when it's challenging to meet all your nutrient needs through food alone. For individuals with dietary restrictions, health conditions that affect nutrient absorption or increased nutritional needs due to aging, supplements can provide essential vitamins, minerals, and other compounds that support health and longevity.

However, it's important to recognize that supplements are not a substitute for a varied and balanced diet. Whole foods offer a complex array of nutrients, fiber, and bioactive compounds that work synergistically to support health in ways that isolated supplements cannot replicate.

Guidelines for Deciding If Supplements Are Right for You

Assess Your Diet and Health: Start by evaluating your diet and health status. Are there nutrients you consistently struggle to obtain from food? Do you have health conditions that might increase your need for certain nutrients?

Consult a Healthcare Professional: Before starting any supplement regimen, consult with a healthcare professional, such as a dietician or a doctor. They can help identify any nutritional deficiencies, recommend appropriate supplements, and ensure that any supplements you take won't interact with medications or existing health conditions.

Consider Your Age and Lifestyle: Certain life stages and lifestyles may increase the need for supplementation. For example, older adults may benefit from vitamin D and calcium supplements for bone health, while vegans might need vitamin B12 and omega-3 supplements.

Suggested Action Steps

Track Your Food Intake

Consider keeping a food diary for a short period. This can be an eye-opening experience, providing insights into your nutritional patterns and helping you identify areas for improvement. Many apps make tracking your intake simple and can offer a breakdown of the nutrients you're consuming, helping ensure a balanced diet.

Experiment with New Foods

One of the most enjoyable aspects of adopting anti-aging nutrition principles is the opportunity to explore and experiment with new foods. Challenge yourself to try at least one new superfood or whole food each week. Whether it's a vegetable you've never cooked with or a grain you've never tasted, each new addition brings its unique blend of nutrients and benefits to your diet.

Gradually Adjust Your Dietary Patterns

Lasting change comes from gradual, consistent efforts. Start by introducing one new anti-aging nutrition principle into your diet at a time. If you're not used to eating leafy greens, for instance, begin by adding a handful of spinach to your smoothies or salads. As these changes become part of your routine, continue to build on them, slowly adjusting your dietary patterns to align more closely with your goals.

Educate Yourself

Knowledge is power, especially when it comes to nutrition. Take time to learn about the benefits of different foods and how they contribute to longevity and vitality. This understanding can make the process more meaningful and motivate you to make informed choices.

Seek Support

Change is easier with support. Share your goals with

friends or family members who might also be interested in adopting healthier eating habits. Joining online communities or forums can also provide encouragement, inspiration, and accountability.

Reflect and Adjust

Regularly reflect on your progress and the changes you've made. What's working for you? What challenges have you encountered, and how can you overcome them? Be prepared to adjust your goals and strategies as needed. Remember, the journey to incorporating anti-aging nutrition principles into your life is on-going and evolving.

By reflecting on your current habits, setting realistic goals, and taking actionable steps, you can gradually embrace a diet that supports ageless vitality. This journey is not just about the foods you eat but about fostering a deeper, more harmonious relationship with your body and its nutritional needs.

Conclusion

As we reach the conclusion of our journey through the principles of anti-aging nutrition, it's important to reflect on the key insights and strategies that can guide us toward a life of vitality and longevity. We've explored the foundational role of whole, unprocessed foods, the importance of balance and variety in our diet, and the critical need for proper hydration. We've delved into the remarkable benefits of superfoods, the longevity secrets of the world's healthiest diets, and practical ways to overcome common nutritional challenges. Moreover, we've discussed the nuanced role of supplements and outlined a week of ageless eating to kickstart this transformative journey.

Recap of Key Points

- **Whole Foods over Processed:** Emphasizing nutrient-dense, whole foods is crucial for combating aging and promoting overall health.
- **Balance and Variety:** A diverse diet ensures a broad spectrum of vitamins, minerals, and antioxidants, supporting cellular health and longevity.
- **Proper Hydration:** Water is essential for every cellular function, aiding in detoxification and maintaining vitality.
- **Superfoods for Ageless Vitality:** Incorporating foods rich in antioxidants and anti-inflammatory properties can significantly impact health and longevity.
- **Dietary Patterns for Longevity:** Adopting dietary habits from cultures known for their longevity, such as the Mediterranean diet, offers a blueprint for healthy living.
- **Overcoming Nutritional Challenges:** With strategic planning and mindful choices, it's possible to navigate busy schedules, dietary restrictions, and budget constraints.
- **Supplements:** While not a substitute for a balanced diet, supplements can fill nutritional gaps when necessary, provided they are chosen with care.

Motivational Closing Thoughts

The journey toward ageless vitality is not merely about extending our years but enriching the quality of every moment we live. Nutrition, with its profound impact on our health, well-being, and longevity, is a powerful tool in this quest. It's a testament to the idea that the choices we make at the dining table can indeed transform our lives, offering a path to a future where every year is met with strength, energy, and a zest for life.

Embrace this journey with an open heart and a spirit of

exploration. Remember, the path to vitality is personal and unique to each individual. It's never too late to make changes that can enhance your health and well-being. With each meal, you have the opportunity to nourish not just your body but your soul, paving the way for a life filled with joy, vitality, and longevity.

Let this be your invitation to a life where age is just a number and vitality is a testament to the power of nutrition.

3

Eternal Movement: Building Strength, Flexibility, and Endurance for Life

This chapter delves into the critical role of physical activity in promoting longevity and vitality. It emphasizes the importance of a balanced approach to exercise that includes strength training, flexibility exercises, and cardiovascular activities.

Introduction to Eternal Movement

The journey toward ageless vitality is not solely nourished by what we eat but also by how we move. Regular physical activity stands as a pillar of health, especially as we age, offering a fountain of youth that flows through every aspect of our well-being. This chapter begins by exploring the myriad benefits of embracing movement in our lives and dispelling common myths that may hinder our path to lifelong fitness.

The Benefits of Regular Physical Activity for Aging Well

Physical activity is a powerful ally in the quest for longevity and vitality. Its benefits permeate every layer of our being, offering not just a longer life, but a richer, more vibrant one. Here are key ways in which regular exercise contributes to aging well:

- **Enhanced Muscular Strength and Bone Density:** Resistance training and weight-bearing exercises fortify muscles and bones, reducing the risk of osteoporosis and falls, common concerns as we age.
- **Improved Flexibility and Balance:** Activities that enhance flexibility, such as yoga and stretching, help maintain mobility, reduce injury risk, and improve the quality of daily life.
- **Boosted Cardiovascular Health:** Aerobic exercises, from brisk walking to cycling, strengthen the heart, lower blood pressure, and improve circulation, combating heart disease, the leading cause of death globally.
- **Mental Health and Cognitive Function:** Exercise is a potent mood enhancer, reducing symptoms of depression and anxiety. Moreover, it has been linked to improved cognitive function, potentially delaying the onset of dementia and Alzheimer's disease.
- **Metabolic Regulation:** Regular movement helps regulate blood sugar levels and has been shown to be a key factor in weight management and the prevention of type 2 diabetes.
- **Increased Longevity:** Beyond preventing disease, physical activity is associated with increased lifespan, adding not just years to life but life to years.

Debunking Myths about Exercise and Aging

Despite the clear benefits, misconceptions about exercise and aging persist, often deterring older adults from engaging in physical activity. Let's address and debunk some of these myths:

- **Myth: It's too late to start exercising.** Reality: It's never too late. Starting exercise at any age can improve health, enhance quality of life, and increase longevity. The body's ability to adapt and grow stronger persists well into older age.
- **Myth: Exercise is dangerous for older adults.** Reality: When tailored to individual capabilities and health conditions, exercise is safe and beneficial for people of all ages. The risks of not exercising far outweigh the carefully managed risks of exercising.
- **Myth: Only high-intensity exercise is beneficial.** Reality: Moderate and low-intensity activities also offer significant health benefits. The key is regularity and finding a form of exercise that is enjoyable and sustainable.
- **Myth: Exercise is only for physical health.** Reality: The benefits of exercise extend well beyond physical health, including significant improvements in mental health, cognitive function, and emotional well-being.

Embracing movement as a cornerstone of aging well invites us to challenge these myths and recognize the transformative power of exercise. By integrating regular physical activity into our lives, we unlock the door to a future marked by vitality, strength and an enduring zest for life.

The Pillars of Physical Wellness

To navigate the path toward ageless vitality, understanding the three pillars of physical wellness—strength training, flexibility exercises, and endurance activities—is essential. Each plays a unique role in fostering a body that not only ages gracefully but also maintains the vigor and resilience needed to enjoy life's myriad adventures.

Strength Training: The Foundation of Youth

Strength training, often perceived as the domain of athletes and bodybuilders, holds profound benefits for individuals of all ages, particularly for those in aging populations. Far from being merely about building muscle mass, strength training is a cornerstone of maintaining youthfulness, vitality, and independence as we age. This section explores the multifaceted benefits of strength training for older adults, outlines simple and safe exercises, and offers tips for seamlessly integrating strength training into your routine.

Benefits of Strength Training for Aging Populations

- **Combating Muscle Loss:** After the age of 30, individuals can lose 3% to 5% of their muscle mass per decade. Strength training reverses this trend, promoting muscle growth and enhancing muscular strength, which are crucial for daily activities and maintaining independence.
- **Boosting Metabolic Rate:** With increased muscle mass comes a higher resting metabolic rate, making it easier to maintain a healthy weight and combat obesity-related diseases.
- **Enhancing Bone Density:** A regular strength training increase bone density and reduces the risk of osteoporosis, a significant concern for older adults, particularly women post-menopause.
- **Improving Balance and Coordination:** By strengthening muscles and joints, strength training reduces the risk of

falls, a leading cause of injury among seniors.

- **Alleviating Symptoms of Chronic Conditions:** Strength training can help manage symptoms of arthritis, back pain, obesity, heart disease, depression, and diabetes, contributing to overall better health and quality of life.

Simple, Safe Strength Training Exercises

1. **Chair Squats:** Stand in front of a chair with feet shoulder-width apart. Lower your body towards the chair as if to sit, then return to standing. This exercise strengthens the legs and core.
2. **Wall Push-Ups:** Stand an arm's length from a wall. Place your hands on the wall at shoulder height and width. Bend your elbows to bring your chest closer to the wall, then push back. This targets the chest, shoulders, and arms.
3. **Seated Leg Lifts:** Sit on a sturdy chair with your feet flat on the ground. Straighten one leg at a time and lift it to knee height. Lower it back down slowly. This exercise strengthens the thighs and abdominal muscles.
4. **Bicep Curls with Light Weights:** Hold a light dumbbell in each hand, arms at your sides, palms facing forward. Bend your elbows to lift the weights towards your shoulders, then lower them slowly. This works the biceps and forearms.
5. **Toe Stands:** Stand behind a chair for support. Slowly rise onto your tiptoes, then lower back down. This strengthens the calves and improves balance.

Tips for Incorporating Strength Training into Your Routine

- **Start Slowly:** Begin with light weights or body weight exercises, gradually increasing the weight and intensity as your strength improves.
- **Focus on Form:** Proper form is crucial to prevent injuries. Consider working with a trainer initially to learn the correct techniques.
- **Be Consistent:** Aim for two to three strength training sessions per week, allowing muscles time to recover between workouts.
- **Listen to Your Body:** If an exercise causes pain, stop immediately. Differentiate between the natural discomfort of muscle exertion and pain that signals an injury.
- **Incorporate Variety:** Vary your exercises to target all major muscle groups and prevent boredom. This will ensure balanced muscle development and maintain your motivation.
- **Set Realistic Goals:** Celebrate progress, whether it's lifting heavier weights, completing more repetitions, or simply feeling stronger in daily life.

Strength training is an invaluable component of an anti-aging regimen, offering a pathway to preserve and enhance physical function, independence, and quality of life. By adopting a tailored, mindful approach to strength training, individuals of all ages can tap into the fountain of youth that lies within the power of their own bodies.

Flexibility: The Key to Lifelong Mobility

Flexibility, often overshadowed by the more visible outcomes of strength and endurance training, plays a crucial role in aging gracefully and maintaining mobility in daily life. As we age, our muscles and joints naturally lose some of their elasticity, leading to decreased range of motion, stiffness, and pain, which can significantly impact the quality of life. This section explores the importance of flexibility for aging populations, highlights effective stretching routines and yoga poses, and offers strategies for incorporating flexibility exercises into everyday routines.

The Impact of Flexibility on Aging and Daily Activities

Flexibility is essential for performing a wide range of daily activities with ease, from bending down to tie shoelaces to reaching for items on a high shelf. As flexibility decreases, these simple tasks can become more challenging and may lead to a reliance on others for basic needs, diminishing independence. Moreover, limited flexibility increases the risk of muscle tears, joint pain, and injuries, as stiff muscles and joints are less capable of absorbing impact and adapting to sudden movements.

Maintaining or improving flexibility through regular stretching can help counteract these age-related changes. It enhances the range of motion, reduces muscle tension, and improves posture, contributing to a more active and pain-free lifestyle. Additionally, flexibility exercises can have a calming effect on the mind, reducing stress and promoting relaxation, which is beneficial for overall well-being.

Stretching Routines and Yoga Poses for Enhanced Flexibility

1. **Dynamic Stretching Routine:** Begin with gentle, dynamic stretches to warm up the muscles. Arm circles, leg swings, and gentle torso twists are excellent for increasing blood flow and preparing the body for more static

stretches.

2. **Static Stretching Routine:** After warming up, move on to static stretches, holding each stretch for 15-30 seconds. Focus on major muscle groups such as the hamstrings, quadriceps, calves, chest, shoulders, and back. Examples include the seated forward bend, standing quadriceps stretch, and chest opener stretches.

3. **Yoga Poses:** Yoga is an effective way to enhance flexibility while also focusing on breathing and relaxation. Poses such as the Cat-Cow Stretch, Downward-Facing Dog, Cobra Pose, and Child's Pose target various muscle groups, improve flexibility, and promote a sense of calm.

Strategies for Integrating Flexibility Exercises into Everyday Life

- **Make It a Routine:** Dedicate a specific time each day for flexibility exercises, such as in the morning to awaken the body or in the evening to wind down before bed.
- **Incorporate Flexibility Breaks:** Take short breaks throughout the day to stretch, especially if you spend long periods sitting. Simple stretches at your desk can alleviate muscle stiffness and improve circulation.
- **Combine Activities:** Incorporate flexibility exercises into activities you already enjoy, such as watching TV or listening to music, to make the practice more enjoyable and sustainable.
- **Set Realistic Goals:** Establish achievable goals related to flexibility, such as being able to touch your toes or comfortably perform a yoga pose that was previously challenging.

- **Seek Guidance:** Consider attending a yoga class or following online tutorials designed for all levels, especially if you're new to flexibility training. This can provide motivation and ensure you're performing stretches safely and effectively.

Flexibility is a vital component of a holistic approach to aging well. By regularly engaging in stretching routines and yoga, individuals can maintain the mobility and independence necessary for a fulfilling life, while also enjoying the mental and emotional benefits that come with a relaxed and flexible body.

Building Endurance: Heart Health and Beyond

Endurance, or the ability to sustain physical activity over time, plays a critical role in cardiovascular health and overall longevity. A strong cardiovascular system ensures efficient delivery of oxygen and nutrients to tissues, supports the removal of waste products, and helps regulate blood pressure and heart rate. This section highlights the importance of cardiovascular health for longevity, suggests low-impact endurance exercises suitable for all ages, and outlines strategies for gradually increasing endurance.

The Importance of Cardiovascular Health for Longevity

Cardiovascular health is foundational to longevity and quality of life. A robust cardiovascular system reduces the risk of heart disease, stroke, and hypertension—conditions that significantly impact morbidity and mortality rates worldwide. Moreover, good cardiovascular health supports cognitive function by ensuring adequate blood flow to the brain, potentially reducing the risk of dementia and cognitive decline. Regular endurance training strengthens the heart muscle, improves circulation, and helps manage weight, contributing to enhanced vitality and extended healthy years.

Low-Impact Endurance Exercises for All Ages

Low-impact endurance exercises are gentle on the joints, making them suitable for individuals of all fitness levels and ages, including those with arthritis or recovering from injury. These exercises effectively improve cardiovascular health while minimizing the risk of stress-related injuries.

1. **Walking:** Brisk walking is accessible, requires no special equipment, and can be easily incorporated into daily routines. It effectively raises the heart rate, improving cardiovascular fitness.
2. **Swimming:** Swimming and water aerobics offer full-body workouts that enhance heart health without putting strain on the joints, making them ideal for older adults or those with joint issues.
3. **Cycling:** Stationary or outdoor cycling is another excellent low-impact option that boosts endurance and cardiovascular health. It can be adjusted for intensity, making it suitable for beginners and seasoned athletes alike.
4. **Elliptical Training:** Using an elliptical machine provides a cardiovascular workout that mimics running but with reduced impact on the knees and hips.
5. **Rowing:** Rowing, whether on water or a rowing machine, is a low-impact, high-reward activity that improves cardio-vascular fitness and strengthens multiple muscle groups.

Gradually Increasing Endurance Through Consistent Practice

Building endurance is a gradual process that requires consistency and patience. Here are strategies to safely increase endurance over time:

- **Start Slow:** Begin with short, manageable sessions and gradually increase the duration and intensity of your workouts. For example, start with 10-15 minutes of continuous activity and slowly build up to 30 minutes or more.
- **Incorporate Interval Training:** Mix short bursts of higher intensity activity with periods of lower intensity. This approach, known as interval training, can significantly improve cardiovascular fitness and endurance.
- **Listen to Your Body:** Pay attention to how your body responds to increased activity. Adequate rest and recovery are essential to prevent overtraining and injury.
- **Set Incremental Goals:** Establish small, achievable milestones to keep motivated. Celebrate progress, such as being able to walk or cycle further without stopping.
- **Stay Consistent:** Regularity is key to building and maintaining endurance. Aim for at least 150 minutes of moderate aerobic activity or 75 minutes of vigorous activity per week, as recommended by health authorities.

Endurance training is not just about enhancing heart health; it's a gateway to improved overall well-being, energy levels, and longevity. By engaging in low-impact endurance exercises and gradually increasing your endurance, you can enjoy the myriad benefits of a strong, healthy cardiovascular system at any age.

Balancing Act: Creating a Well-Rounded Exercise Routine

Achieving ageless vitality and maintaining optimal health

as we age require a holistic approach to physical activity. A well-rounded exercise routine that incorporates strength training, flexibility exercises, and endurance activities offers a comprehensive strategy for enhancing physical wellness. This balanced approach ensures that we're not just focusing on one aspect of fitness but nurturing our bodies in a way that promotes overall health, mobility, and longevity. Here, we explore guidelines for developing such a balanced exercise plan and discuss the crucial role of rest and recovery in sustaining a lifelong fitness regimen.

Guidelines for Developing a Balanced Exercise Plan

1. **Incorporate All Three Pillars:** Ensure your weekly exercise routine includes elements of strength training, flexibility exercises, and endurance activities. This combination supports muscle health, joint mobility, cardiovascular fitness, and overall well-being.
2. **Start with a Solid Foundation:** Begin each workout session with a warm-up that includes dynamic stretching to prepare your muscles and joints for the activity ahead. This can help prevent injuries and improve performance.
3. **Strength Training:** Aim for at least two strength training sessions per week, focusing on major muscle groups. Utilize bodyweight exercises, free weights, or resistance bands. Ensure you're challenging your muscles while still being able to maintain proper form.
4. **Flexibility Exercises:** Dedicate time for flexibility exercises or yoga at least two to three times per week. These sessions can be on your rest days or after a strength or endurance workout. Focus on stretching all major muscle groups, holding each stretch for 15-30 seconds.

5. **Endurance Activities:** Incorporate moderate to vigorous aerobic activities into your routine on most days of the week, aiming for a total of at least 150 minutes of moderate-intensity or 75 minutes of high-intensity aerobic physical activity, as recommended by health guidelines.

6. **Listen to Your Body:** Pay attention to how your body responds to different types of exercises and adjust your routine accordingly. If you're feeling fatigued or experiencing discomfort, consider modifying the intensity or duration of your workouts.

7. **Vary Your Routine:** Keep your exercise regimen interesting by varying your activities. This not only prevents boredom but also challenges your body in new ways, promoting continued improvement and reducing the risk of plateaus.

The Role of Rest and Recovery

Rest and recovery are as integral to a fitness regimen as the exercises themselves. They allow your body to heal, adapt, and strengthen in response to the physical demands placed on it.

- **Scheduled Rest Days:** Incorporate at least one to two rest days per week to allow muscles to repair and grow. Rest days are also important for mental rejuvenation and motivation.

- **Active Recovery:** Consider light activities such as walking, gentle yoga, or stretching on rest days. Active recovery can help maintain mobility while still allowing your body to recover.

- **Adequate Sleep:** Ensure you're getting enough quality sleep each night. Sleep is crucial for muscle recovery, hormonal balance, and overall health.

- **Hydration and Nutrition:** Support your body's recovery process with proper hydration and a balanced diet rich in nutrients. Protein, in particular, is essential for muscle repair and growth.

A well-rounded exercise routine that balances strength, flexibility, and endurance training with adequate rest and recovery is key to achieving and maintaining optimal health and vitality at any age. By following these guidelines, you can create a sustainable fitness regimen that supports lifelong wellness and enables you to enjoy a vibrant, active life.

Making Exercise Enjoyable

Ultimately, the key to making exercise a regular and enjoyable part of life is to approach it with a positive attitude and an open mind.

- **Mix It Up:** Variety not only keeps things interesting but also challenges your body in new ways, enhancing overall fitness.
- **Reward Yourself:** Set up a reward system for meeting your fitness goals. Rewards could be a relaxing massage, a new book, or anything that feels like a treat.
- **Reflect on the Benefits:** Regularly remind yourself of the benefits you're gaining from exercise, such as improved mood, increased energy, and better health. This can help keep the bigger picture in focus and make exercise feel more like a gift to yourself than a task.

By addressing these common barriers with practical strategies, you can transform exercise from a daunting obligation into a valued and enjoyable part of your daily life, paving the way for a healthier, more active future.

Tailoring Your Approach: Exercise at Any Age

Adapting exercise routines to align with the evolving needs and abilities of our bodies through different life stages is crucial for maintaining optimal health, vitality, and quality of life. As we age, our physical capabilities, health status, and fitness goals naturally change, necessitating adjustments to our exercise regimens. This section explores how to adapt exercise routines across various life stages, with special considerations for older adults, ensuring that physical activity remains a beneficial and integral part of life at any age.

Adapting Exercise Routines through Life Stages

- **Youth and Adolescence:** Focus on establishing a foundation of regular physical activity that includes a mix of aerobic, strength, and flexibility exercises. Encourage participation in sports, dance, or martial arts to foster a positive relationship with exercise and build social connections.
- **Adulthood:** As work and family commitments increase, finding time for exercise can be challenging. Prioritize efficient, balanced workouts that combine elements of strength, flexibility, and endurance. High-intensity interval training (HIIT) can be particularly effective for those short on time.
- **Middle Age:** Pay attention to the body's changing needs, incorporating more low-impact endurance activities like cycling or swimming to reduce stress on joints. Strength

training becomes increasingly important to counteract muscle loss and metabolic slowdown.

- **Senior Years:** Focus on exercises that maintain or improve balance, flexibility, and bone density, such as tai chi, yoga, and light resistance training. Endurance activities should be low-impact, with walking and water aerobics being excellent choices.

Special Considerations for Exercise in Older Adults

- **Consult Healthcare Providers:** Before starting or modifying an exercise routine, older adults should consult with healthcare providers, especially if they have existing health conditions. This ensures that exercise plans are safe and tailored to individual health needs.
- **Emphasize Balance and Flexibility:** Incorporating balance and flexibility exercises is crucial for preventing falls, a common risk for older adults. Practices like yoga or tai chi not only improve balance but also enhance mental well-being.
- **Adjust Intensity and Duration:** Older adults may need to adjust the intensity and duration of their workouts. Starting with shorter, less intense sessions and gradually increasing as fitness improves can help prevent injury and encourage adherence.
- **Incorporate Social Activities:** Group classes or walking groups can provide social support, making exercise more enjoyable and sustainable. Social connections are also beneficial for mental health.
- **Monitor and Adapt:** Regularly assess how the body responds to exercise routines and be willing to adapt

based on comfort, performance, and enjoyment. Flexibility in approach allows for sustained activity and benefits throughout the aging process.

Exercise is a lifelong journey that should evolve with us, offering benefits that extend far beyond physical health. By tailoring exercise routines to meet the changing needs and abilities of each life stage, with special attention to the unique considerations of older adulthood, we can ensure that movement remains a joyous and integral part of our lives, from youth through to our senior years.

Conclusion: Movement as a Way of Life

As we conclude our exploration of the vital role of physical activity in fostering ageless vitality, it's important to reflect on the journey we've undertaken together. From understanding the foundational pillars of physical wellness—strength, flexibility, and endurance—to recognizing the importance of a balanced exercise routine and the necessity of rest and recovery, we've charted a course toward a more vibrant and fulfilling life. We've addressed common barriers to movement and outlined strategies for tailoring exercise to meet the evolving needs of our bodies through every stage of life. Moreover, we've delved into the significance of setting realistic goals, tracking progress, and finding motivation through community, personal rewards, and a focus on the myriad benefits of exercise.

Recap of Key Points

- **The Pillars of Physical Wellness:** Strength training, flexibility exercises, and endurance activities each play a unique role in maintaining and enhancing our physical health as we age.

- **Balancing Act:** Developing a well-rounded exercise plan that incorporates all three pillars is essential for achieving ageless vitality.
- **Rest and Recovery:** Integral to a lifelong fitness regimen, allowing our bodies to heal and grow stronger.
- **Overcoming Barriers:** Practical solutions for common challenges like time constraints, lack of motivation, and fear of injury can make exercise a regular and enjoyable part of life.
- **Exercise at Any Age:** An adapting exercise routine to meet changing needs ensures that physical activity remains a constant, beneficial presence throughout our lives.
- **Measuring Progress and Staying Motivated:** Essential strategies for maintaining momentum and ensuring that our fitness journey continues to move forward.

Inspirational Closing Thoughts

Embracing physical activity is not merely about extending our years but enriching the quality of every day we live. It's about discovering strength we didn't know we had, enjoying flexibility in body and mind, and feeling the exhilarating rush of endurance that carries us through life's challenges. Movement is a celebration of what our bodies can do, a testament to the resilience and adaptability that define the human spirit.

As we move forward, let us remember that movement is more than a routine—it's a way of life. It's the rhythm to which our bodies were born to move, a melody of muscles stretching and contracting, of hearts beating strong and sure. In every step, every stretch, every lift, we find a deeper connection to ourselves and the world around us.

Let physical activity be your companion on the journey toward ageless vitality. Let it be the thread that weaves through the tapestry of your days, adding color, texture and vibrancy. And as you embrace movement as a cornerstone of your life, may you discover not just the joy of motion but the profound satisfaction of knowing you are living your life to its fullest, most vibrant potential.

4

The Sleep Revolution: Restoring Energy through Deep, Healing Sleep

This chapter delves into the transformative power of sleep, a fundamental yet often undervalued component of ageless vitality. It explores the science behind sleep and its profound impact on health, well-being, and longevity. Through understanding the mechanisms of restorative sleep, addressing common sleep challenges, and adopting practices that promote deep, healing rest, readers can unlock the door to rejuvenated energy and enhanced life quality.

Introduction to the Sleep Revolution

In the tapestry of human health and vitality, sleep is the thread that weaves together our physical well-being, mental clarity, and emotional resilience. Often overlooked in the hustle of daily life, sleep remains one of the most powerful, yet underappreciated, pillars of health. This chapter embarks on a journey to uncover the transformative power of sleep, highlighting its indispensable role in nurturing a life of ageless vitality and dispelling the myths that cloud our understanding of sleep, especially as we age.

The Critical Role of Sleep

Physical Health: Sleep is the foundation upon which our body repairs, rebuilds, and rejuvenates. It plays a pivotal role in immune function, with adequate rest being crucial for the body to fight off infections and diseases. During sleep, the body undergoes processes that repair muscle tissue, synthesize proteins, and regulate hormones responsible for growth and appetite, directly impacting our physical strength, weight management, and overall health.

Mental Clarity: The brain uses sleep to consolidate memories, process information, and clear out toxins that accumulate during waking hours. This nightly reset enhances cognitive functions, including learning, problem-solving, and decision-making, ensuring that we remain sharp, focused, and mentally agile.

Emotional Resilience: Sleep deeply influences our emotional and psychological well-being. It helps regulate mood, reduce stress, and improve our capacity to cope with daily challenges. Adequate sleep is associated with better emotional regulation, reduced risk of depression and anxiety, and a more positive outlook on life.

Debunking Common Myths About Sleep and Aging

Myth 1: Older adults need less sleep. While sleep patterns may change with age, the need for restorative sleep remains constant. Older adults require as much sleep as younger adults—7 to 8 hours per night—to maintain optimal health and cognitive function.

Myth 2: Waking up during the night means poor sleep quality. It's normal for sleep architecture to change with age, including more frequent awakenings. However, these do not necessarily indicate poor sleep quality, as long as one can return to sleep and complete the sleep cycles needed for restorative rest.

Myth 3: Daytime napping is a sign of laziness or poor health. Strategic napping can be a valuable tool for supplementing night time sleep, especially if night sleep is disrupted. Short naps can enhance alertness and well-being without necessarily indicating health issues.

Myth 4: Insomnia and sleep problems are just part of aging. While more common in older adults, sleep disturbances like insomnia are not an inevitable part of aging and can often be addressed through lifestyle changes, sleep hygiene practices, or medical intervention if necessary.

Embracing the sleep revolution means recognizing the profound impact that sleep has on our lives and debunking the myths that prevent us from prioritizing this critical aspect of health. As we delve deeper into the science and strategies for enhancing sleep, we open the door to a world of rejuvenated energy, sharper minds, and resilient spirits, laying the foundation for a life of ageless vitality.

How Sleep Patterns Change with Age and the Implications

As we age, our sleep architecture undergoes significant changes, which can affect our overall health and vitality:

- **Altered Sleep Structure:** Older adults tend to spend more time in the lighter stages of sleep (non-rapid eye-movement (NREM) Stage 1 and 2) and less time in deep sleep (NREM Stage 3) and Rapid eye movement (REM) sleep. This shift can impact the restorative quality of sleep, affecting physical recovery and memory consolidation.

- **Increased Sleep Fragmentation:** Aging is often accompanied by more frequent awakenings throughout the night. These disruptions can reduce sleep efficiency, leading to daytime sleepiness and affecting overall quality of life.
- **Shifted Sleep Patterns:** Many older adults experience advanced sleep phase syndrome, where they feel sleepy earlier in the evening and wake up earlier in the morning. This shift can interfere with social activities and personal preferences, impacting mental well-being.
- **Greater Susceptibility to Sleep Disorders:** Conditions such as insomnia, sleep apnea, and restless legs syndrome are more prevalent in older populations, further complicating the ability to achieve restful sleep.

Understanding these changes is crucial for adapting our sleep habits and environments as we age. By acknowledging and addressing the evolving nature of our sleep patterns, we can take proactive steps to mitigate their impact on our health and vitality, ensuring that sleep remains a rejuvenating and restorative force throughout our lives.

The Impact of Sleep on Health and Longevity

Sleep, an essential yet often neglected component of our daily lives, plays a pivotal role in maintaining and enhancing our health and longevity. Its influence extends far beyond merely resting the body, deeply impacting our immune function, cognitive health, emotional well-being, and metabolic processes. Understanding the multifaceted impact of sleep can illuminate why prioritizing restorative rest is crucial for a life of vitality and wellness.

Sleep and Immune Function

The relationship between sleep and the immune system is a dynamic interplay where both influence each other significantly. During sleep, the body produces and releases cytokines, a type of protein that targets infection and inflammation, effectively creating an immune response. Sleep deprivation can decrease the production of these protective cytokines, as well as antibodies and cells that fight off infections, making us more susceptible to illnesses and prolonging recovery times. Adequate sleep, therefore, is essential for bolstering the body's defenses against infectious diseases and supporting the effectiveness of vaccines.

Sleep's Role in Cognitive Health and Memory Consolidation

Sleep is paramount for cognitive processes, including learning, memory consolidation, problem-solving, and decision-making. During sleep, particularly in the deep stages, the brain processes and consolidates memories from the day. This is when short-term memories are transferred to long-term storage, making space for new information. Furthermore, sleep facilitates the removal of toxins in the brain that accumulate during waking hours, including beta-amyloid, a protein associated with Alzheimer's disease. Thus, consistent, quality sleep is a cornerstone of cognitive health, helping to maintain mental clarity and protect against cognitive decline.

The Connection between Sleep, Mood Regulation, and Mental Health

There's a profound link between sleep and our emotional and psychological well-being. Lack of sleep can affect the brain's regulation of emotions, leading to increased irritability, stress, and susceptibility to anxiety and depression. Conversely, adequate sleep helps to regulate mood, enhance resilience to stress, and improve overall mental health. The restorative power of sleep on the mind is akin to hitting a reset button, allowing for emotional balance and stability.

How Adequate Sleep Contributes to Weight Management and Metabolic Health

Sleep plays a significant role in regulating metabolic functions, including the hormones that control appetite: ghrelin (which signals hunger) and leptin (which signals fullness). Sleep deprivation can lead to an imbalance in these hormones, increasing hunger and appetite, often for high-calorie, carbohydrate-rich foods. Additionally, poor sleep can impact the body's ability to regulate blood sugar and increase the risk of type 2 diabetes. Adequate sleep supports healthy weight management and metabolic health by maintaining hormonal balance, reducing cravings, and enhancing the body's natural metabolic processes.

In conclusion, the impact of sleep on health and longevity is profound and far-reaching. By prioritizing sleep, we support our body's immune function, protect and enhance cognitive health, regulate mood and emotional well-being, and maintain metabolic health. Embracing the full spectrum of sleep's benefits is essential for anyone looking to lead a life marked by vitality, resilience, and longevity.

Common Sleep Challenges and Their Solutions

In the quest for restorative sleep, many individuals encounter obstacles that can hinder their ability to achieve deep, healing rest. From insomnia and disrupted sleep patterns to sleep apnea and the impact of lifestyle choices, these challenges can significantly affect one's quality of life. Understanding these common sleep issues and implementing effective strategies for improvement can pave the way to better sleep and, consequently, better health.

Insomnia and Disrupted Sleep Patterns

Causes: Insomnia can stem from a variety of sources, including stress, anxiety, hormonal changes, and medical conditions. Disrupted sleep patterns may also result from poor sleep hygiene, such as irregular sleep schedules, and the use of electronic devices before bedtime.

Effects: Insomnia and irregular sleep patterns can lead to daytime fatigue, difficulty concentrating, mood disturbances, and a decreased quality of life. Over time, chronic sleep deprivation may contribute to more serious health issues, such as heart disease, diabetes, and obesity.

Strategies for Improvement:

- **Establish a Regular Sleep Schedule:** Going to bed and waking up at the same time every day can help regulate your body's internal clock.
- **Create a Relaxing Bedtime Routine:** Activities such as reading, taking a warm bath, or practicing relaxation techniques can signal to your body that it's time to wind down.
- **Limit Exposure to Screens:** The blue light emitted by phones, tablets, and computers can interfere with melatonin production, making it harder to fall asleep. Try to avoid screens at least an hour before bedtime.
- **Manage Stress:** Techniques such as mindfulness medita-

tion, deep breathing exercises, and journaling can reduce stress and anxiety, promoting better sleep.

Sleep Apnea and Other Sleep Disorders

Recognition and Understanding: Sleep apnea is characterized by pauses in breathing during sleep, leading to disrupted sleep and decreased oxygen levels. Other common sleep disorders include restless legs syndrome and narcolepsy. Recognizing the symptoms, such as loud snoring, daytime sleepiness, and sudden awakenings, is the first step toward management.

Path to Management:

- **Consult a Healthcare Professional:** If you suspect you have a sleep disorder, seek evaluation from a sleep specialist. Diagnosis may involve a sleep study.
- **Adopt Healthy Lifestyle Changes:** Weight loss, avoiding alcohol before bedtime, and sleeping on your side can help manage sleep apnea symptoms.
- **Use Prescribed Therapies:** Treatments such as Continuous Positive Airway Pressure (CPAP) machines for sleep apnea or medication for restless legs syndrome can significantly improve sleep quality.

The Impact of Lifestyle Choices on Sleep Quality

Diet, Exercise, and Screen Time: Consuming caffeine or heavy meals close to bedtime can disrupt sleep, as can a lack of physical activity during the day. Excessive screen time, especially before bed, can also impair sleep quality.

Strategies for Improvement:

- **Mind Your Diet:** Avoid caffeine and heavy, rich foods within a few hours of bedtime. Opt for a light snack if you're hungry.
- **Incorporate Regular Exercise:** Engaging in regular physical activity can help you fall asleep faster and enjoy deeper sleep, but try to avoid vigorous exercise close to bedtime.
- **Limit Screen Time:** Establish a digital curfew to give your brain time to unwind and produce melatonin, the sleep hormone.

Addressing common sleep challenges requires a multifaceted approach that includes lifestyle adjustments, stress management, and, when necessary, medical intervention. By understanding the causes and implementing targeted strategies, individuals can overcome these obstacles, paving the way for deep, restorative sleep and enhanced overall well-being.

Strategies for Enhancing Sleep Quality

Achieving restorative sleep is essential for health and vitality, but it often requires more than just closing our eyes. The environment in which we sleep, our routines leading up to bedtime, and the methods we use to relax can significantly impact the quality of our rest. Here are strategies to enhance sleep quality by focusing on creating a conducive sleep environment, establishing a pre-sleep routine, and utilizing relaxation techniques.

Creating a Sleep-Conducive Environment

Light: Exposure to light plays a crucial role in regulating our circadian rhythms. To foster a sleep-friendly environment, minimize light exposure in the evening. Use blackout curtains or a sleep mask to block out external light, and dim or turn off indoor lights an hour before bedtime.

Noise: A quiet environment is essential for uninterrupted sleep. If you cannot control external noise, consider using earplugs, a white noise machine, or a fan to create a consistent, soothing background sound that masks disruptive noises.

Temperature: The ideal temperature for sleep is around 60-67°F (15-19°C). A room that's too hot or too cold can disrupt sleep, so adjust your thermostat, bedding, and sleepwear to find a comfortable sleep temperature.

The Importance of a Pre-Sleep Routine

Establishing a pre-sleep routine signals to your body that it's time to wind down and prepare for sleep. This routine can include:

- **Dimming the Lights:** Lowering light levels in the evening can help increase the production of melatonin, the hormone that regulates sleep.
- **Limiting Screen Time:** Avoid screens at least an hour before bed to reduce exposure to blue light, which can interfere with sleep.
- **Engaging in Calming Activities:** Reading, listening to soft music, or taking a warm bath can relax the mind and body, making it easier to fall asleep.

A consistent pre-sleep routine not only improves sleep quality but also enhances your ability to fall asleep quickly.

Relaxation Techniques and Mindfulness Practices

Deep Breathing: Slow, deep breathing can reduce stress

and promote relaxation. Try the 4-7-8 technique: inhale for 4 seconds, hold for 7 seconds, and exhale for 8 seconds.

Progressive Muscle Relaxation: This involves tensing and then relaxing each muscle group in the body, starting from the toes and moving up to the head. It reduces physical tension and promotes a sense of calm.

Mindfulness Meditation: Focusing on the present moment can help clear the mind of worries and stress. Guided meditation apps or simply paying attention to your breath can be effective ways to practice mindfulness before bed.

Visualization: Imagining a peaceful scene or a happy memory can divert your mind from stressors and ease you into sleep.

Incorporating these strategies into your nightly routine can significantly enhance the quality of your sleep. By creating a conducive sleep environment, establishing a calming pre-sleep routine, and utilizing relaxation techniques, you can improve not only your sleep but also your overall health and well-being, paving the way for a life filled with energy and vitality.

Addressing Sleep in Different Life Stages

Sleep, an essential component of overall health and well-being, has requirements that evolve throughout our lifespan. Each stage of life brings its own set of challenges and needs regarding rest. Understanding and adapting to these changes can help maintain optimal sleep quality and ensure the restorative rest needed for health and vitality. This section explores how sleep practices can be tailored to meet the changing needs across different life stages, with a focus on special considerations for sleep in older adults.

Tailoring Sleep Practices across the Lifespan

Infants and Children: Young children and infants need significantly more sleep than adults to support their rapid mental and physical development. Establishing regular naps and bedtime routines, creating a quiet and comfortable sleep environment, and limiting screen time before bed can help promote healthy sleep habits early on.

Teenagers: The shift in circadian rhythms during adolescence often pushes teenagers towards later sleep and wake times. Encouraging consistent sleep schedules, even on weekends, and reducing exposure to screens and caffeine in the evening can help teens get the 8-10 hours of sleep they need for growth, learning, and development.

Adults: For working-age adults, balancing the demands of work, family, and social obligations with the need for sleep can be challenging. Prioritizing sleep as a non-negotiable component of health, maintaining a consistent sleep schedule, and creating a wind-down routine before bed are crucial for sustaining energy and well-being.

Special Considerations for Sleep in Older Adults

As we age, changes in sleep architecture, such as increased wakefulness during the night and earlier wake times, become more common. These changes, along with health conditions and medications that can affect sleep, pose new challenges for older adults. However, quality rest remains as important as ever for maintaining cognitive function, emotional balance, and physical health.Top of Form

Measuring Progress and Adjusting Strategies

In the pursuit of restorative sleep and the myriad benefits it brings to health and vitality, it's essential to monitor progress and remain flexible in adjusting strategies as needed. Two critical components in this process are maintaining a sleep diary and understanding when it's appropriate to seek professional help. These tools can empower individuals to take control of their sleep health, identify patterns and issues, and make informed decisions about their sleep practices.

Keeping a Sleep Diary: Tracking Patterns, Disturbances, and Improvements

A sleep diary is a valuable tool for anyone looking to improve their sleep quality. By recording details about your sleep habits, environmental factors, and daily routines, you can uncover patterns and behaviors that either contribute to restful sleep or detract from it. Here's what to include in your sleep diary:

- **Sleep and Wake Times:** Note the time you go to bed, how long it takes you to fall asleep, the number of awakenings during the night, and the time you finally wake up in the morning.
- **Sleep Quality:** Record how you feel upon waking up and throughout the day. Are you rested, or do you feel fatigued?
- **Daytime Habits:** Include information about your caffeine and alcohol consumption, exercise routines, and any naps taken during the day.
- **Environmental Factors:** Note the bedroom temperature, noise levels, and any use of electronic devices before bed.

Over time, this diary will reveal insights into how your behaviors and environment affect your sleep, allowing you to make targeted changes to enhance sleep quality.

When to Seek Professional Help: Recognizing the Signs

While many sleep challenges can be addressed with changes to sleep hygiene and lifestyle, there are instances when consulting a sleep specialist is necessary. Recognizing the signs that professional help is needed is crucial for addressing underlying sleep disorders or health issues that could be impacting your sleep. Consider seeking professional help if you experience:

- **Persistent Insomnia:** Difficulty falling or staying asleep that lasts for several weeks or longer, despite attempts to improve sleep habits.
- **Excessive Daytime Sleepiness:** Feeling overwhelmingly tired during the day, which can indicate sleep disorders such as sleep apnea or narcolepsy.
- **Frequent Nighttime Awakenings:** Regularly waking up during the night and having trouble falling back asleep.
- **Unusual Behaviors:** Actions such as sleepwalking, night terrors, or severe restlessness that disrupt sleep.
- **Snoring and Breathing Issues:** Loud snoring accompanied by gasping or choking sounds, which may suggest sleep apnea.

A sleep specialist can conduct a thorough evaluation, which may include a sleep study, to diagnose and treat any underlying conditions. Treatment options can significantly improve sleep quality and, by extension, your overall health and well-being.

Monitoring your sleep through a diary and being proactive in seeking professional help when necessary are key steps in achieving and maintaining the deep, restorative sleep essential for ageless vitality. These strategies empower individuals to take charge of their sleep health, making adjustments as needed to ensure that sleep remains a rejuvenating and life-enhancing activity.

Conclusion: Embracing the Sleep Revolution

As we conclude our exploration of "The Sleep Revolution," we've journeyed through the essential realms of understanding sleep's profound impact on our health, the common challenges that can disrupt our rest, and the strategies we can employ to enhance the quality of our sleep. This chapter has underscored the critical role of sleep in maintaining physical health, mental clarity, emotional resilience, and overall vitality. We've delved into the science of sleep, highlighting the importance of its stages and cycles, and how our sleep patterns evolve with age. We've addressed the common hurdles to restful nights, from insomnia to sleep apnea, and provided practical solutions for overcoming these obstacles. Moreover, we've outlined actionable steps for cultivating sleep hygiene practices that promote restorative rest, emphasizing the significance of a conducive sleep environment, a pre-sleep routine, and the mindful incorporation of naps.

Recap of Key Points

- **Understanding Sleep:** Recognizing the stages of sleep and their contributions to health sets the foundation for appreciating sleep's complex role in our well-being.
- **The Impact of Sleep:** Sleep is intricately linked with immune function, cognitive health, mood regulation, and metabolic balance, highlighting its importance across all facets of health.
- **Common Sleep Challenges:** Identifying and addressing issues such as insomnia, sleep apnea, and the effects of lifestyle choices on sleep are crucial steps toward better

rest.

- **Strategies for Enhancing Sleep Quality:** From optimizing our sleep environment to establishing calming pre-sleep routines and employing relaxation techniques, we have the power to improve our sleep.
- **Sleep Hygiene:** Adhering to best practices for sleep, including maintaining regular sleep schedules and understanding the interplay between diet, exercise, and rest, is essential for lifelong vitality.
- **Tailoring Sleep Practices:** Adapting our approach to sleep as we navigate different life stages ensures that our rest evolves to meet our changing needs.

Inspirational Closing Thoughts

Embracing the sleep revolution is about more than just understanding the mechanics of sleep; it's about recognizing sleep as a transformative power that can elevate our existence. In the realm of sleep lies the potential for healing, for rejuvenation, and for tapping into the wellspring of vitality that sustains us through the challenges and triumphs of life. As we commit to nurturing our sleep, we unlock the door to ageless vitality, to days filled with energy and purpose, and to a life where every moment is enriched by the quality of our rest.

Let this exploration of sleep inspire you to prioritize your rest as diligently as you do other aspects of your health. Remember, in the quiet of the night, as the world around us falls into slumber, we are given a precious opportunity to reset, to restore, and to revitalize our bodies and minds. By embracing the principles of the sleep revolution, we step into a brighter, more vibrant future, where the dreams of today become the vitality of tomorrow.

Here's to the transformative power of sleep, to the nights that offer healing and the days that brim with the vitality born of restful slumber. May we all find our path to restorative rest and, in doing so, unlock the full potential of our ageless vitality.

5

Mind over Matter: Stress Reduction and Mental Clarity for a Vibrant Life

This chapter delves into the critical relationship between mental well-being and overall health, emphasizing the importance of managing stress and enhancing mental clarity for a life filled with vitality and purpose. It explores the science behind stress and its effects on the body and mind, offers practical strategies for reducing stress, and provides guidance on cultivating mental clarity and resilience.

Introduction to Mind over Matter

In the intricate dance of life, the harmony between mind and body plays a pivotal role in determining our overall health and vitality. This chapter, "Mind over Matter," delves into the profound interconnectedness of mental and physical health, shedding light on how the state of our mind can significantly influence our bodily well-being and vice versa. It also explores the insidious nature of chronic stress, a pervasive issue in modern society, and its far-reaching impacts on both the body and mind. Understanding this relationship is the first step toward cultivating a life marked by resilience, clarity, and vibrant health.

The Interconnectedness of Mental and Physical Health

The bond between mental and physical health is undeniable and complex. Our thoughts, emotions, and mental states can trigger physical responses and conditions, illustrating the body's inherent wisdom and the mind's powerful influence over it. For instance, positive emotions and a calm mind can bolster immune function, enhance heart health, and promote healing and longevity. Conversely, mental distress can manifest physically, leading to a host of health issues, including increased inflammation, disrupted sleep patterns, and heightened susceptibility to illness. This bidirectional relationship underscores the importance of nurturing both mental and physical health in unison, as neglecting one can adversely affect the other.

Chronic Stress: A Modern Malady

Chronic stress, a condition characterized by a prolonged state of physiological arousal in response to persistent stressors, has become a hallmark of contemporary life. Unlike acute stress, which is a natural and necessary response to immediate threats, chronic stress lingers, keeping the body in a constant state of alert. This relentless activation of the stress response system can wreak havoc on the body and mind, leading to a plethora of adverse effects:

- **Physical Health:** Chronic stress can impair the immune system, making the body more susceptible to infections and diseases. It can increase the risk of heart disease, hypertension, and diabetes by promoting unhealthy lifestyle choices and directly affecting cardiovascular and metabolic functions. Additionally, it can exacerbate or contribute to the development of gastrointestinal issues, chronic pain, and sleep disturbances.

- **Mental Health:** The psychological toll of chronic stress is equally concerning. It is a significant risk factor for anxiety, depression, and cognitive decline. Chronic stress can impair memory and concentration, reduce mental clarity, and diminish one's ability to make sound decisions. Over time, it can lead to feelings of burnout, detachment, and a decreased sense of personal accomplishment.

Recognizing the profound impact of chronic stress on both the body and mind is crucial for taking proactive steps toward mitigating its effects. By embracing strategies for stress reduction and mental clarity, individuals can foster a harmonious balance between mind and body, paving the way for a life of enhanced well-being and ageless vitality. This chapter aims to equip readers with the knowledge and tools necessary to navigate the challenges of modern life with resilience and grace, ensuring that the mind and body work together as allies in the pursuit of health and happiness.

The Effects of Stress on Health and Vitality

Stress, particularly when chronic, casts a long shadow over our health and vitality, affecting every aspect of our well-being. Its pervasive influence extends from our physical health, weakening the immune system and compromising heart health, to our mental state, where it becomes a significant factor in conditions such as anxiety, depression, and cognitive decline. Moreover, stress entrenches itself in a vicious cycle with sleep disruption, further exacerbating its effects. Understanding these impacts is crucial for developing strategies to mitigate stress and preserve our health and vitality.

Physical Health

Immune System: Chronic stress takes a toll on the immune system, impairing its ability to fight off antigens and making the body more susceptible to infections and illnesses. The stress hormone cortisol can suppress the effectiveness of the immune system by lowering the number of lymphocytes available. Over time, this diminished immune response can lead to more frequent infections and a slower recovery process.

Heart Health: The relationship between stress and heart health is significant. Stress increases heart rate and blood pressure, putting additional strain on the heart. Over prolonged periods, this heightened state can contribute to inflammation in the cardiovascular system, a risk factor for heart disease and stroke. Additionally, stress-related behaviors such as overeating, physical inactivity, and smoking further increase the risk of cardiovascular problems.

Chronic Disease Risk: Beyond its immediate effects, chronic stress is a contributing factor to the development of several chronic diseases, including obesity, diabetes, and hypertension. Stress can influence behaviours and factors that increase disease risk, such as poor eating habits, lack of physical activity, and smoking. Moreover, the physiological changes induced by stress, including elevated levels of cortisol and adrenaline, can directly contribute to disease processes.

Mental Health

Anxiety and Depression: Chronic stress is a well-known

trigger for anxiety and depression. The constant feeling of being under pressure can lead to feelings of hopelessness and despair, hallmarks of depression. Similarly, the perpetual alertness required in a state of stress can heighten anxiety levels, creating a state of heightened worry and tension.

Cognitive Decline: Prolonged exposure to stress hormones can also affect cognitive functions. High levels of cortisol can impair memory and inhibit the growth of new neurons in the hippocampus, an area of the brain essential for learning and memory. Over time, this can lead to difficulties with concentration, memory, and decision-making.

The Vicious Cycle of Stress and Sleep Disruption

Stress and sleep disruption form a vicious cycle, each exacerbating the other. Stress can make it difficult to fall asleep and stay asleep, leading to a night of restless, unsatisfying sleep. In turn, inadequate sleep can heighten stress levels by reducing the body's ability to cope with stressors, impairing emotional regulation, and decreasing cognitive function. This cycle can become self-perpetuating, with stress leading to poor sleep, which in turn leads to more stress.

Breaking the cycle of stress and its detrimental effects on health and vitality requires a multifaceted approach, including lifestyle changes, stress management techniques, and, when necessary, professional support. By addressing the root causes of stress and developing healthy coping mechanisms, individuals can mitigate its impacts and enhance their overall well-being.

Practical Strategies for Stress Reduction

In the face of life's inevitable stressors, equipping ourselves with effective strategies for stress reduction is essential for maintaining health, vitality, and a sense of well-being. Mindfulness and meditation, physical activity, and adept time management and prioritization emerge as powerful tools in this endeavor, each offering a pathway to tranquility and resilience. Here's how these practices can help mitigate stress and enhance our quality of life.

Mindfulness and Meditation

Techniques for Grounding and Centring the Mind: Mindfulness and meditation are practices that bring your attention to the present moment, helping to break the cycle of rumination and worry that often accompanies stress. Techniques include:

- **Focused Attention Meditation:** Choose a focus point, such as your breath or a mantra and gently bring your attention back to it each time your mind wanders. This practice helps cultivate a state of calm and focus.
- **Body Scan Meditation:** Lie down or sit comfortably and mentally scan your body from head to toe, noticing any areas of tension or discomfort. This can help connect you to your physical self and release stored stress.
- **Mindful Walking:** Take a walk and focus on the experience of walking, paying attention to the sensations in your feet and the rhythm of your steps. This combines the benefits of mindfulness and gentle physical activity.

Incorporating mindfulness and meditation into your daily routine, even for just a few minutes a day, can significantly reduce stress levels and improve mental clarity.

Physical Activity as a Stress Reliever

The Role of Exercise in Reducing Cortisol Levels and Improving Mood: Engaging in regular physical activity is one of the most effective ways to combat stress. Exercise reduces levels of the body's stress hormones, such as adrenaline and cortisol, and stimulates the production of endorphins, the body's natural painkillers and mood elevators. Activities can include:

- **Aerobic Exercise:** Activities like walking, running, cycling, or swimming increase heart rate and can significantly reduce stress, improve sleep, and boost overall mood.
- **Strength Training:** Lifting weights or using resistance bands can alleviate stress by focusing the mind on the task at hand and away from stressors.
- **Yoga and Tai Chi:** These practices combine physical movement, breath control, and meditation, offering a holistic approach to stress reduction.

Finding an activity you enjoy and making it a regular part of your routine can provide an outlet for stress and enhance your sense of well-being.

Deepening Mindfulness and Meditation Practices

To deepen the impact of mindfulness and meditation on stress reduction, consider integrating these practices into routine activities beyond designated meditation times. For instance:

- **Mindful Eating:** Turn meals into an exercise in mindfulness by eating slowly, savoring each bite, and paying attention to the flavours, textures, and sensations of your food. This practice can enhance digestion and satisfaction with meals while reducing stress-related eating habits.

- **Mindful Communication:** Practice active listening and mindful speaking in your interactions. This can improve relationships, reduce misunderstandings, and lower stress levels associated with social interactions.

Expanding Physical Activity Options

While aerobic exercise, strength training, and practices like yoga are foundational, exploring diverse forms of physical activity can keep your routine engaging and effective in stress reduction:

- **Nature Walks:** Spending time in nature has been shown to lower stress levels, improve mood, and enhance mental well-being. Incorporate walks in natural settings into your exercise routine to reap these benefits.
- **Dance:** Dancing combines physical activity with creative expression, making it an enjoyable way to relieve stress and improve mood. Whether in a class or your living room, dancing can lift spirits and reduce tension.
- **Team Sports:** Participating in team sports can offer a sense of community and support, alongside the physical benefits of exercise. The social interaction involved can further contribute to stress reduction.

Refining Time Management and Prioritization

Enhancing your time management and prioritization skills can involve adopting new tools and techniques that fit your lifestyle and preferences:

- **Digital Tools:** Utilize apps and digital planners for organizing tasks, setting reminders, and tracking deadlines. Many tools offer features that can help prioritize tasks and manage time more effectively.

- **Mind Mapping:** Use mind mapping for complex projects or when you're feeling particularly overwhelmed. This visual form of organizing thoughts and tasks can help clarify priorities and actionable steps.
- **Scheduled Downtime:** Just as you schedule work tasks and appointments, schedule regular intervals of downtime. These periods are essential for mental recovery and can increase productivity and creativity in the long run.

By embracing and integrating these strategies into your life, you're not just reducing stress; you're investing in a foundation of practices that support mental clarity, emotional resilience, and physical health. This holistic approach to managing stress not only enhances your ability to navigate the challenges of daily life but also contributes to a deeper sense of fulfillment and vitality. Remember, the journey to mastering stress and cultivating a vibrant life is ongoing and ever-evolving, reflecting the dynamic nature of our needs and circumstances.

Enhancing Mental Clarity

Mental clarity is the cornerstone of effective decision-making, creativity, and overall well-being. It allows us to navigate the complexities of life with confidence and purpose, making it essential for achieving our full potential. This section explores the significance of mental clarity, introduces cognitive exercises and activities to maintain and enhance mental sharpness and discusses the critical role of diet and nutrition in supporting brain health and cognitive function.

The Importance of Mental Clarity

Decision-Making: Mental clarity enables us to assess situations accurately, weigh options logically, and make informed decisions. It cuts through the fog of overwhelm and indecision, allowing for choices that align with our values and goals.

Creativity: A clear mind is a fertile ground for creativity. It fosters an environment where innovative ideas can flourish, unencumbered by the clutter of unrelated thoughts and worries. Mental clarity enhances our ability to connect disparate ideas and envision novel solutions.

Overall Well-Being: Beyond its impact on decision-making and creativity, mental clarity contributes to emotional balance and stress reduction. It helps us maintain perspective, manage challenges with equanimity, and cultivate a sense of inner peace.

Cognitive Exercises and Activities

To promote mental sharpness and focus, consider incorporating the following cognitive exercises and activities into your routine:

- **Brain Games:** Puzzles, word games, and strategy-based games challenge the brain, improve problem-solving skills, and enhance cognitive flexibility.
- **Learning New Skills:** Taking up a new hobby or learning a new language stimulates the brain, encourages neural growth, and can improve memory and focus.
- **Mindful Reading:** Engaging with complex texts or literature not only provides new knowledge but also enhances comprehension skills, attention span, and critical thinking.

Building Emotional Resilience

Emotional resilience is the ability to adapt to and recover from stress, adversity, and life's challenges. It's a crucial skill that enables individuals to navigate the ups and downs of life with grace and strength. Developing a resilient mind-set, nurturing positive relationships, and learning from setbacks are foundational components of building emotional resilience. Here's how to cultivate these aspects in your life for enhanced emotional strength and well-being.

Conclusion: Embracing a Life of Mental Clarity and Resilience

As we conclude our exploration of "Mind over Matter," we've journeyed through the landscapes of stress reduction, mental clarity, and emotional resilience. This chapter has illuminated the profound impact that mastering our mental and emotional well-being has on our lives, offering practical strategies and insights for navigating life's challenges with grace and strength. We've delved into understanding stress and its effects, highlighted the importance of mental clarity for decision-making and creativity, and outlined the pillars of building emotional resilience. Here, we recap the essential strategies for cultivating a vibrant inner life and offer some closing thoughts on the transformative journey ahead.

Recap of Key Points

- **Understanding Stress:** Recognizing the biological under-pinnings of stress and differentiating between acute and chronic stress are foundational steps in managing its impact on our lives.
- **Practical Strategies for Stress Reduction:** Techniques

such as mindfulness and meditation, physical activity, and effective time management and prioritization have been identified as powerful tools for mitigating stress and enhancing well-being.

- **Enhancing Mental Clarity:** We explored cognitive exercises and the role of diet and nutrition in supporting brain health, emphasizing the importance of mental clarity for overall vitality.
- **Building Emotional Resilience:** Developing a resilient mindset, nurturing positive relationships, and learning from setbacks are key to navigating life's ups and downs with emotional strength and flexibility.
- **Integrating Stress Reduction into Daily Life:** Creating a personal stress management plan and the importance of regular self-reflection and adjustment ensure that stress reduction becomes a seamless part of our daily routine.

Inspirational Closing Thoughts

The journey to mastering one's mind is perhaps the most profound and rewarding adventure we can undertake. It's a path that leads not only to improved health and reduced stress but to a deeper sense of fulfillment and purpose in life. By embracing the strategies outlined in this chapter, we unlock the potential to transform our lives from the inside out, cultivating a state of mental clarity and emotional resilience that radiates through every aspect of our being.

This transformative power holds the key to navigating the complexities of the modern world with ease and confidence, allowing us to meet each moment with a clear mind and a resilient heart. As we continue to practice and integrate these principles into our lives, we discover that the true essence of vitality and fulfillment lies in our ability to master our inner landscape.

Let this chapter serve as a beacon, guiding you toward a life where stress is managed with grace, challenges are met with resilience, and every day is infused with clarity and purpose. Remember the journey to mastering your mind is on-going, filled with opportunities for growth, learning and profound personal transformation. Embrace this journey with an open heart and a curious spirit and watch as your life unfolds in ways more vibrant and fulfilling than you ever imagined. Here's to your journey of mental clarity and resilience—a journey that shapes not just your own life but the world around you.

6

The Power of Connection: Cultivating Social Bonds for Longevity and Happiness

This chapter delves into the essential role of social connections and relationships in promoting longevity and enhancing happiness. It explores the science behind social bonds, their impact on health and well-being, and practical strategies for nurturing meaningful relationships in our lives.

Introduction to the Power of Connection

Human beings are inherently social creatures, wired for connection from the moment we enter the world. This fundamental need for social interaction is not just a matter of emotional fulfillment but is deeply intertwined with our physical health, mental well-being and overall longevity. The bonds we form with others—whether they are family, friends or community members—serve as a vital source of support, joy and meaning in our lives.

The Fundamental Human Need for Social Connection

Our drive for social connection is rooted in survival. Early humans who formed strong social bonds were more likely to thrive, as cooperation increased their chances of finding food, protecting each other, and caring for offspring. Today, while we may not face the same survival challenges, the need for connection remains, influencing our behaviour, choices, and well-being in profound ways.

Overview of How Social Bonds Influence Physical Health, Mental Well-Being and Longevity

Physical Health: Social connections have a significant impact on our physical health. Strong social ties have been linked to a lower risk of numerous health issues, including heart disease, high blood pressure, and weakened immune function. People with robust social networks tend to have better health outcomes, recover faster from surgery, and even live longer.

Mental Well-Being: The quality of our relationships also deeply affects our mental and emotional health. Social support can buffer against stress, reduce the risk of depression and anxiety, and enhance feelings of self-worth and belonging. Conversely, loneliness and social isolation can exacerbate mental health issues and diminish life satisfaction.

Longevity: Perhaps most strikingly, research has shown that strong social connections can increase longevity. A meta-analysis of studies found that individuals with strong social relationships have a 50% increased likelihood of survival, regardless of age, gender, health status, and cause of death, underscoring the life-extending power of social bonds.

The Science of Social Connections

Research Findings on the Health Benefits of Strong Social Ties

Studies across various disciplines consistently demonstrate the health benefits of strong social ties. These benefits range from reduced inflammation and lower blood pressure to improved immune response. Socially connected individuals also tend to adopt healthier lifestyles, further contributing to their well-being.

The Impact of Loneliness and Social Isolation on Health Risks and Mortality

Conversely, loneliness and social isolation have been identified as significant health risks, comparable to smoking, obesity, and physical inactivity. Loneliness can increase cortisol levels, elevate blood pressure, and weaken the immune system, making individuals more susceptible to a range of diseases. Moreover, the emotional pain of feeling disconnected can lead to depression, anxiety, and cognitive decline, highlighting the critical need to nurture our social connections for a healthy, fulfilling life.

In sum, the science of social connections reveals a clear picture: the relationships we cultivate profoundly impact our health, happiness, and how long we live. As we delve deeper into the power of connection, we uncover not only the roots of our social nature but also the pathways through which we can enrich our lives and the lives of those around us.

Social Bonds and Physical Health

The intricate web of social connections we weave throughout our lives plays a pivotal role in shaping our physical health. From the health of our hearts to the robustness of our immune systems and our ability to manage stress, the quality and depth of our relationships can have profound implications. Furthermore, social support not only aids in recovery from illness but also serves as a preventive measure against a host of diseases.

How Relationships Affect Heart Health, Immune Function and Stress Levels

Heart Health: Social bonds can significantly impact heart health, with strong relationships associated with lower risks of cardiovascular diseases. Positive social interactions can help lower blood pressure and reduce the risk of heart disease by providing emotional support, encouraging healthier lifestyle choices, and offering a buffer against stress, which is a known risk factor for heart conditions.

Immune Function: Our social connections also influence our immune system's effectiveness. People with vibrant social lives tend to have stronger immune responses. The support offered by relationships can lead to lower levels of stress hormones like cortisol, which, when chronically elevated, can suppress immune function. Moreover, positive social interactions can boost the production of protective substances like antibodies, enhancing the body's ability to fend off infections and illnesses.

Stress Levels: The presence of supportive relationships acts as a buffer against stress. Knowing that one has a reliable social network can lessen the perceived severity of stressful situations, leading to lower stress responses. This reduction in stress is not only beneficial for mental well-being but also mitigates the physical wear and tear on the body associated with chronic stress, such as inflammation and hormonal imbalances.

The Role of Social Support in Recovery from Illness and Disease Prevention

Recovery from Illness: Social support plays a crucial role in the recovery process from illness or surgery. Individuals with strong support networks often experience better recovery outcomes, attributed to both the practical aspects of having help with daily tasks and the emotional support that fosters a positive outlook and adherence to treatment plans. The encouragement and care provided by loved ones can significantly impact one's motivation to recover and maintain health.

Disease Prevention: Beyond aiding recovery, social connections can act as a preventive measure against various diseases. The emotional support, companionship, and sense of belonging provided by social ties can encourage healthier lifestyle choices, such as regular exercise, a balanced diet, and adherence to medical advice. Additionally, the stress-reducing effect of good relationships lowers the risk of conditions exacerbated by stress, including hypertension and metabolic syndrome.

In essence, the bonds we form and maintain throughout our lives are not just a source of joy and fulfillment; they are foundational to our physical health. By nurturing these connections, we not only enrich our lives with meaningful interactions but also fortify our bodies against the challenges of illness and stress, paving the way for a healthier, more vibrant existence.

Social Connections and Mental Wellbeing

The fabric of our social connections intricately weaves through the tapestry of our mental well being, offering strength, color, and texture to the overall picture of our health. The quality and depth of our relationships play a pivotal role in buffering against mental health conditions and enhancing our happiness, life satisfaction, and resilience. This section explores the vital link between social bonds and mental wellbeing, highlighting how meaningful relationships contribute to a fortified mind and a fulfilled life.

The Role of Technology in Social Connections

Tips for Using Technology to Enhance Rather Than Replace Face-to-Face Interactions

To harness the benefits of technology while mitigating its drawbacks, consider the following tips:

- **Be Intentional with Social Media Use:** Use social media platforms to facilitate real-world connections, such as organizing events, sharing meaningful content, or reaching out to friends for in-person meetups. Avoid mindless scrolling and focus on interactions that deepen relationships.
- **Quality Over Quantity:** Prioritize meaningful, quality interactions over the quantity of connections. A few close, supportive relationships are more beneficial than a large number of superficial contacts.
- **Set Boundaries:** Create boundaries around device use, especially during social gatherings. Designate tech-free times or zones where the focus is on engaging with the people around you, fostering deeper connections.
- **Leverage Technology for Deepening Connections:** Use video calls to maintain long-distance relationships, allowing for face-to-face conversations that convey nonverbal cues and emotions. Share photos, videos, or messages that spark deeper discussions and mutual interests.
- **Digital Detoxes:** Regularly unplug from digital devices

to recharge and refocus on personal interactions. Periodic digital detoxes can help reset your relationship with technology and encourage more meaningful engagement with others.

By thoughtfully integrating technology into our lives, we can enhance our social connections, bridging the gap between digital convenience and the irreplaceable value of face-to-face interactions. Technology, when used wisely, can be a powerful tool for nurturing and sustaining the deep, meaningful relationships that are essential for our well-being and happiness.

Conclusion: Embracing the Power of Connection

As we conclude our exploration of "The Power of Connection," we've journeyed through the profound impact of social bonds on our physical health, mental well-being, and overall happiness. This chapter has illuminated the essential role that relationships play in enhancing our quality of life, offering practical strategies for nurturing these connections in the modern world. We've delved into the science of social connections, the benefits of strong social ties, and the challenges and opportunities presented by technology in maintaining meaningful relationships. Here, we recap the essential insights and offer some closing thoughts on the transformative power of social bonds.

Recap of Key Points

- **The Fundamental Human Need for Connection:** Social bonds are not just beneficial but essential for our health and happiness, deeply rooted in our evolutionary past.

- **Impact on Physical Health and Longevity:** Strong relationships contribute to better heart health, stronger immune function, and reduced stress levels, ultimately leading to longer, healthier lives.
- **Enhancement of Mental Well-Being:** Social connections buffer against mental health conditions like depression and anxiety, fostering happiness, life satisfaction, and resilience.
- **Building and Maintaining Relationships:** In the digital age, it's crucial to cultivate meaningful relationships through intentional social media use, community involvement, and prioritizing face-to-face interactions.
- **Navigating Relationship Challenges:** Addressing common barriers such as time constraints and technological distractions, and employing techniques for effective communication and conflict resolution, are key to sustaining healthy relationships.
- **The Role of Technology:** While technology presents challenges, it also offers opportunities to enhance connections when used thoughtfully, emphasizing the importance of complementing digital interactions with in-person experiences.

Inspirational Closing Thoughts

The journey through "The Power of Connection" reaffirms the transformative potential of social bonds in our lives. As we navigate the complexities of the modern world, let us remember that at the heart of our well-being lies the simple yet profound act of connecting with others. These connections, whether with family, friends, or the wider community, are the threads that weave the rich tapestry of our lives, imbuing them with color, warmth, and vibrancy.

Embracing the power of connection means more than just building a network of relationships; it's about deepening those bonds, sharing our joys and sorrows, and supporting each other through life's ups and downs. It's about recognizing our shared humanity and the strength that comes from knowing we are not alone.

As we move forward, let us commit to fostering these essential connections, for they hold the key to a life filled with longevity, happiness, and fulfilment. Let the power of connection illuminate our path, guiding us toward a future where every individual feels valued, supported, and connected. Here's to embracing the transformative potential of social bonds, for in connection, we find the essence of what it means to be truly alive.

7

The Path Forward: Integrating Ageless Vitality into Your Life

The journey toward ageless vitality is both personal and universal, a series of choices and commitments made in the pursuit of well-being. It is a path marked by continuous learning, adaptation, and growth, guided by the understanding that vitality is not merely the absence of disease but the presence of health, joy, and a deep engagement with life. Here are key considerations for integrating the principles of ageless vitality into your life:

- **Embrace Holism:** Recognize that vitality encompasses physical, mental, emotional, and social well-being. Each aspect of health influences and supports the others, forming a holistic framework for living fully. Strive for balance, nurturing each dimension of your well-being with equal care and intention.
- **Cultivate Mindfulness:** Approach your health journey with mindfulness, staying present and attentive to your body's needs, your emotional state, and your relationships.

Mindfulness enhances your connection to the moment, empowering you to make choices that align with your goals for vitality.

- **Adopt Flexibility:** Be open to adjusting your strategies as your needs and circumstances evolve. Ageless vitality is not a static goal but a dynamic process of adaptation and growth. What works for you today may need refinement tomorrow, and that's okay.
- **Foster Community:** Remember the power of connection and community in supporting your journey. Share your experiences, seek support when needed, and offer encouragement to others. The journey toward vitality is enriched by companionship and shared wisdom.
- **Prioritize Consistency:** Small, consistent actions over time yield significant results. Whether it's choosing nutritious foods, engaging in regular physical activity, practicing stress reduction techniques, or connecting with loved ones, consistency is key to integrating ageless vitality into your life.
- **Celebrate Progress:** Acknowledge and celebrate your achievements, no matter how small. Each step forward is a victory in the journey toward a more vibrant, fulfilling life. Celebrating progress fosters motivation and reinforces your commitment to ageless vitality.

Inspirational Closing Thoughts

The path to integrating ageless vitality into your life is both a challenge and a profound opportunity—an opportunity to rediscover the joy of living, to embrace each day with energy and purpose, and to cultivate a deep sense of fulfilment. As you embark on this journey, let the principles explored in this exploration serve as your guide, illuminating the way toward a life marked by health, happiness, and a vibrant engagement with the world around you.

Remember, ageless vitality is not just a destination but a way of being, a choice to live each moment with intention and grace. It's a commitment to nurturing yourself, body, mind, and spirit, and to sharing the light of your vitality with others. Here's to your journey toward ageless vitality—a journey that unfolds with each breath, each choice, and each day lived to its fullest potential.

www.ingramcontent.com/pod-product-compliance
Lightning Source LLC
Chambersburg PA
CBHW051834250726
48659CB00005B/1835